Dressing to Look Younger

A 15 Minute Guidebook To Help You Look Younger Than Ever

Lisa Lewis

PUBLISHED BY:

Lisa Lewis

Table of Contents

Introduction

Aging is inevitable and no one is immune to it. A way to maintain constant youth is to go for surgical procedures and to buy tons of cosmetics that promise eternal youth.

Not everybody has the money or the time to spend on cosmetic procedures or to test all the beauty products that may not even work. We have therefore compiled this report to help you with ways on how to look younger by dressing correctly.

This guide will help you look younger without looking immature, to dress in a more youthful manner, but still maintain the grace and sophistication of your age. It will help you identify the frequent fashion mistakes and guide you to good style in fashion.

At the very least it will convince you that there are alternatives to cosmetic procedures that are pricey and invasive. It will convince you that beauty does not have to know pain and that you have a lot to gain, but without the pain.

Chapter 1: Know Your Body Type and What Styles to Avoid

Not every person is born with the perfect body type. In fact, even super models each have a unique body type. Knowing your body type will help you to choose styles that will make you look younger by complimenting your body type. Men and woman each have different categories to which their body types are identified.

Women's body types

Women's body types can be classified into the following categories:

- **Pear Body Shape**

Definition

Women with pear shaped bodies have hips, thighs and bottoms that are wider that their shoulders. Their upper bodies are smaller than the lower body and they tend to have flat stomachs.

Styles to choose

Best styles for a pear shaped woman, would be clothing that emphasises your upper body. Choose slim fitted tops, bold and bright shirts, shirts with large collars and sleeves, cardigans and shirts with buttons. Choose a shirt or jersey with an embellished neckline or with a halter neck top.

The main idea is to focus the attention upwards to the slimmer part of the body. Use this to add detail and modern styles to create a younger image. An A-line dress is classic and the latest dresses comes in modern version of the classic style. The A-line dress places emphasis on your upper body while also slimming down the wider hips of the pear shaped body.

Another way to draw attention to your upper body is to layer your clothes. Not only does it divert attention to your upper body, it is also in fashion and a trend to add youth to your appearance.

When choosing pants, choose pants with wider legs. The wider hems balance out with your hips and visually create a slimmer image. Tailored pants are a good option to buy according to your body shape. A bootleg pants will also work as the flare at the bottom will add width to balance with your hips.

For shoes you can consider pointed shoes and sandals with heels, as this elongates your legs, especially when worn with wide legged pants.

Wear jewellery around your neckline to draw attention to it. Stockings in a neutral colour can be worn to smooth out the appearance of your legs, but it is important to note that it has to be neutral colours, or at least a colour that does not clash with your shoes.

When looking to buy swimsuits, the same principal applies: you need to buy a swimsuit that will add volume to your upper body and create an illusion of broader shoulders. Also look for bottoms that will not put emphasis on your lower body.

To create the illusion of broader shoulders, opt for tops with straps that are set wide apart and of which the straps are broad. Go for light coloured tops with patterns or trimmings on it. The bottom part of the swimsuit should cover your bottom completely or at least moderately. Try a bottom that has scoop or high-cut legs as this will make your legs look slimmer and longer.

Styles to avoid

Style to avoid would be any style that places emphasis on your lower body. These fashions include pencil skirts, tube skirts or any tight fitting skirts.

Flashy pants like cargo pants should be avoided, not only because it will draw attention to you lower body, the pocket features on the pants will actually add width and bulk to your hips and thighs. Tapered pants should also be avoided

Avoid shoes with rounded toes as it will make your legs look stomped off. When wearing stockings, the colour of the stockings should not clash with your shoes, as clashing colours will give the leg a segmented appearance and draw attention to your lower body.

Other names

Although *Pear shape* is the most common name for this body type, it is also known by the following descriptions:

- Bell Shape

- A-shape (Upward triangle)

There are really no differences in body shape for the above description.

- **Spoon body shape**

Definition

The spoon body type is much like a pear shape body type where the hips are wider than the shoulders, but you have a defined waist. Despite the defined waist, the spoon shaped women's body are more likely to develop "love-handles" at her waist and also she is more inclined to gain weight in her stomach. The spoon shape lady usually has very shapely arms and lower leg.

Styles to choose

The important rule for spoon shaped figures is again to divert attention from your weakest asset, your lower body, to your best asset, your upper body. Less emphasis should be drawn to your stomach to create the illusion of balance and to create the illusion of an hour glass figure.

Tops should be chosen with patterns or designs that will create a balance with your lower body. It should accentuate your waist, but should cover and camouflage your tummy bulges if you have any.

Wear tops that have an empire waist, or other tops that slim your waist down without adding more volume. Tops that are strapless or off the shoulder will draw attention to your shoulders and add width to it, creating balance. Also wear tops with V or U necks or ruching detail around your bust.

For women with a spoon shaped figure, their legs are one of their best assets, so choose bottoms that will accentuate your legs. Wear A-line skirts or dresses and experiment with mini-skirts.

Pants should have a straight leg, not flared, and wear pants that are solid colours and where a wide waist-band to camouflage your mid-section of bulges.

With swimsuits, if you are buying a one piece, go for a high waist pin up style piece or one with ruching at the waist.

For a two piece, mix and match pieces. Wear a light coloured top with padding, patterns or ruffle detail and match it with a darker coloured bottom.

For both one piece and two pieces, find a swimsuit of which the straps of the top are in the middle of your shoulders.

Styles to avoid

As with pear shapes bodies, avoid pants and skirts that are tight fit.

Avoid styles that draw attention to your lower body such as tapered pants, cargo and harem styled pants.

Pants should not be multi coloured and bold patterned either.

Tops should not draw attention to your tummy, but rather to your waist, so avoid vest styled tank tops.

- **Hourglass body shape**

Definition

The hourglass figure is the ideal figure, as the hips and bust are proportionally the same width and you have a define waist. Your shoulders are gently rounded and aligned perfectly with your hips. You have a perfect side and front profile with balance and harmony.

Styles to choose

To make the most of your hourglass figure, you should wear clothes that will keep your hips and shoulders in balance and accentuate your waistline. By adding a bit of detail either to your upper body or hips, you can add more volume to create the illusion of curves. Wide belts worn over shirts and dresses help to accentuate your waist.

Skirts of any length can be worn with an hourglass figure as your legs are one of your best features and you can experiment with different styles.

Any tops that will add focus to your defined waist can be worn such as belted tops and tops with banding at the waist. Tailored tops and jackets that are form fitting, as well as wrap-style tops are good choices.

The hourglass figured woman has no limitations to pants, but the best choices for pants are pants with a boot cut or a straight leg pants. High wasted pants will accentuate your slim waistline.

The rule with an hourglass figure is really to always create balance, so whether you are wearing a skinny or tight fit pant, or if you are wearing cargo pants, always wear a top that balances out the pants.

Choosing a swimsuit style should be no problem as any style suits an hourglass figure as long as it is balanced and proportioned evenly. You may want to opt for a padded top to add volume to your bust, or a straight cut bottom to create a more slimming effect.

When choosing a top with straps, the straps should be midway over your shoulders to keep the proportion to your hips.

Styles to avoid

With the hourglass figure there are no styles to avoid. What you should remember though is to keep the proportions balanced between your hips, waist and shoulders.

Wear proportionally matched pants or skirts and top to keep your perfect image.

- **Straight Body Type**

Definition

This body type is also known as rectangle or rule shape and is the most common body shape. Your hips, waist and upper body are not well defined ad creates the image of a straight line. A woman with this body shape usually has very shapely legs and tends to gain weight at her upper body and arms.

Styles to choose

When choosing clothes for straight figured women, choose clothing pieces that will create volume and definition to your waist and to your upper body, but that will enhance your waist and create an hourglass illusion.

This should be done proportionally to keep a balanced image.

Tailored tops that are taken in at the waist or with a belt are good choices to add definition to your waist. A top with a ruche or embellished effect at the bust will create an illusion of a bigger bust. V neck and U neck tops will also draw attention to your upper body.

Off shoulder tops or tops with structured shoulders and sleeves will create an image of broader shoulders.

Pants and skirts should add volume and curves to your hips. Mid-rise or low-rise pants with wide waistbands draws attention to your hips, making it look curvier. Pant with full legs or moderately flared legs are also good choices. Choose detail on the pants such as pockets that flap or are embellished to create volume.

Full skirts or tiered skirts of any length can be worn, but experiment with mid-length skirts, or mini-skirts to show your shapely legs.

Mid-length skirts will create a subtle segmented image to place more definition on your waist.

With swimsuits you can choose any suit that will create more volume at your bust and also draw more attention to your shoulders, such as a swimsuit with wide-set straps. Light coloured tops and tops that are padded, embellished and ruffled will help create more curves.

Bottoms can also be light coloured, but opt for a bottom with a waistband to define your waist.

- **Top Hourglass**

Definition

A top hourglass figure is a well-defined figure, much like the standard hourglass figure. The waist, hip and bust ratio is curvaceous, but the bust is larger than the hips. Your legs are shapely and one of your best assets. Your bottom should be more rounded than flat, creating a front and side profile that is balanced and in harmony.

Styles to choose from

Women with top hourglass figures can wear any styles, but they need to focus on either slimming down their bust, or to create more volume at their hips.

This can be achieved by wearing V neck shirts and tops that are narrower at the waist. Also choose a tailored shirt or jacket. Dark coloured tops will slim down the bust area.

For bottoms, you can choose pants with a bootleg or semi-flared legs to give width to your hips. Cargo pants or pants with pockets will have the same effect.

A full skirt or A-line skirt flatters a top hourglass figure, but also wear mini-skirts to flaunt your shapely legs.

For accessories, consider hip belts or a scarf worn as a belt over your hips for a modern style that also adds width to your hips.

When buying a swimsuit, apply the same rule as with your clothes. Balance out your upper body with your lower body. Opt for darker, solid color tops and lighter, patterned bottoms. Halter neck tops paired with a frilled or embellished bottom makes a good match. You can also choose a straight cut bottom that goes over your hips.

- **Inverted Triangle body type**

Definition

The most prominent feature of an inverted triangle body type is the large shoulders and upper body in proportion to the lower body. This body type has slim hips and subtle waist and very broad shoulders and wide back. Your legs should be your best feature.

Styles to choose

To create a balance between your upper body and lower body, it is important for the inverted triangle body type to slim down your shoulders and back and to add volume to your hips and lower body. Also try to accentuate your waist more.

Choose wrap style tops or tops with a narrow V necks. Tops that are narrowed down at the waist will define your waist better. Tailored tops and jackets are always a good choice to add style and definition to any body type. Wear darker colored tops to slim down your shoulders.

Bottoms should be chosen to add volume to your lower body, so choosing wide legged pants will work to balance out your hips. Boot cut pants will add width to your legs. Pants with flap pocket detail are effective to give volume to your hips and create balance to your figure.

Skirts styles for the inverted triangle figure, is a full A-line skirt in lighter colours, and even with selective patterns on.

Your swimsuit should also be mixed pieces where you combine a detailed bottom with a plain and slimming top. The tops should be dark coloured and the bottom lighter coloured or patterned. Bottoms with ruffles or side details will also create an illusion of fuller hips.

Accessories to choose will be waist belts to define your waist, or hip belts to add volume to your hips. Heeled shoes will elongate your legs, but choose a round toed shoe to add a wider illusion to balance your hips.

- **Oval body type**

Definition

Oval body types are characterised by narrow hips, a large midsection and waist, and a large, full bust. The waist is the largest part of your frame, and also undefined. These body types are also identified by a full face and short, full neck. Their best assets are their legs.

Styles to choose

The most important rule to remember with the oval body type is that your waist needs to be defined and less emphasis should be placed on your mid-section. To achieve this image, you have to wear clothes that get tapers at the waist.

Wear tops that are V neck and wear wrap style shirts and jackets. Tops that flare at the bottom are excellent to add width to your hips and slim down the midsection.

Full skirts will create balance with your shoulders and you can experiment with lengths to emphasise your legs. Be careful not to wear skirts that are too short as it will increase the oval look of your midsection. Skirts that flare and bubble skirts will also work for a balanced look.

Choose wide-legged pants and flared pants as this will add width to your hips. Pants with flap pockets on the side will draw attention to your hips. Use this to your advantage and wide waistbands to your look.

When choosing a swimsuit, choose a suit that will add definition to your waist. One piece suits with an hourglass print is a good option, so are bikinis with a tank top. Go for swimsuits that crisscross or wrap. Match pieces such as light colored tops with bottoms that have detail at the hips, such as ties.

Styles to avoid

Avoid any style that will add more emphasis to your midsection like tops with horizontal stripes and tops with bold patterns around the midsection.

Avoid too short skirts and flat shoes with stomped off toes as it will make your profile also look stomped off.

- **Diamond body shape**

This body type is characterised by hips being broader than your bust and shoulders, and a full midsection. The widest part of the diamond frame, is the midsection, and the waist is undefined.

Styles to choose

Clothing for the diamond figured needs to be chosen to slim down your midsection, slim down your hips, define your waist and also to enhance your upper body.

Tops that taper towards your waist. Also wear belted tops to slim your midsection and add volume to your hips.

Choose clothes that will add curves where needed, such as wearing a pants with wide or flared legs and a wide waistband. Wear dark colored bottoms to create a slimming effect and wear pant with pocket details at the back and sides.

When wearing a skirt, opt for A-line skirts, or skirts that are lightly gathered. A full length skirt is always a classic, but be aware not to wear a too short skirt. Your legs may be flaunted, but wearing a too short skirt will make you look stomped off.

Do wear high heels with your skirts and pants to add length and slim down your mid-section.

Finding a suitable swimsuit, the same rules apply as for the oval shaped women. Find suits that define your midsection and that will also divert attention away from your midsection. The best option is to mix darker colored tops on wide set shoulder items. Bottoms may be colored and details added to the waist to create a fuller image. Tank top bikinis will slim down your waist line and define your hips.

- **Conclusion**

After reviewing all this information, there are a few basic rules that must be adhered to when dressing to make you look younger.

- Create balance. Divert focus away from parts that need less emphasis and add more emphasis to less prominent areas to create balance in you hip, waist and bust proportions.

- Darker and plain fabric slims down

- Lighter and patterned fabric creates volume

- Horizontal lines create width

- Vertical lines create length

- Pointed heeled shoes creates length

- Round toe flat shoes decreases length

Men's body types

Body types for men are categorised differently from women's body types. The body types for men are as follows:

- **Ectomorph**

Definition

An ectomorph man has a lean build. He is slender and small of frame with a flat chest. They usually have thin and narrow shoulders thin limbs and stringy muscles. They have difficulty to pick up weight and they have a fast metabolism.

Fashion to choose

Even though the ectomorph body are slender, wearing clothes with a proper fit is very important. Avoid wearing clothes that are too tight fit or skinny clothes as it will make you look anorexic and malnourished.

Clothes that fit too loosely, will not create the appropriate youth illusion, it will in fact make you look like a young boy and immature.

Dress shirts, t-shirts and blazers are good choices to wear. Wear it in lighter colors to add volume. Polo neck shirts will add focus to your neck and create width.

Avoid darker colours, especially wearing a bottom and top in a dark colour as it will take away volume and make you look leaner.

- **Mesomorph**

Definition

A mesomorph body type is an athletic type with a large bone structure and large muscles. Men with this body type are well-built, or at least their bone and muscle structure allows for an athletic frame with a tendency to broader shoulders and a narrower waist.

To balance out the shoulders, men with a mesomorph body type should wear straight cut or wide leg pants.

For shirts, choose shirts with a wide cut shoulders, but narrows down to your hips to accentuate your waist. Jackets should be hip length or mid-thigh length. Choose natural material and natural stretch material and not made from elasticised fabrics as it tends to cling to your body and not fit naturally.

Avoid patterns on your clothes, but if you do wear patterns, opt for smaller patterns.

Wear well fitted clothes and do not wear baggy clothes. You do not want to hide your athletic frame, and besides, baggy clothes can very easily create a neglected image.

- **Endomorph**

Definition

The endomorph body type is basically the opposite of ectomorph. They tend to be more solid and less lean than the ectomorph. They have a more rounded body frame. They have a shorter build, but have strong muscles, especially in their legs. They also tend to have thicker legs and arms.

Styles to choose

Wear shirts that will emphasise your shoulders and divert attention away from your stomach. Dark colored shirts will create a leaner image. If you want to wear a patterned shirt, wear one with vertical lines to elongate your upper body and create a more defined waist.
Choose pants with a waistband that goes over the waist. Don't wear pants of which the waistline is too small and fits under your stomach as this will make your stomach look larger and your legs thinner and

shorter. Avoid tight fitting pants and skinny pants as it will add more volume to your waist.

- **Combination body types**

<u>Definition</u>

It is not uncommon for men to have a combination of these body types. Combination body types are ectomorph / mesomorph and mesomorph / endomorph. These body types are a specific body type, but display characteristics of another body type. A typical example is an ectomorph body type that has a slower metabolism than usually expected and tend to gain weight easier than a true ectomorph.

<u>Styles to choose</u>

Styles should be chosen according to your primary body type, but needs to be adjusted at problem areas to draw attention away from that area and place more emphasis on your better features.

Chapter 2: Factors That Are Aging You

Certain styles can add many years to your appearance. Avoid the following styles if you do not want to age pre-maturely due to your clothes. Rather wear the more youthful options if you have no other choice but to wear these styles.

Boring-Belt Syndrome

When wearing a belt to create a younger image, wear the belt as an accenting feature point. It should have aesthetic value, not just functionality. Do away with boring belts that are used to keep your pants up. Rather adjust the size of your pants for a better fit.

For a more youthful image, wear belts in different styles and colours. Wear thin belts with dark trousers and choose a belt color that contrasts with the trouser. Thick belts work well with dresses, cardigans and jackets. When worn correctly, it can create a slimmer image to your waist.

Choose styles of belts that work with every outfit such as shimmery belts, brown leather belts and animal print belts.

Silk-Scarf Syndrome

We all know the silk scarf. The little scarf Grandma and Aunt Annie used to wear and all the women in the community on Sundays during church. Unfortunately that image is imprinted and stuck in our minds. So, sad to say, the moment you tie a silk scarf around your neck or drape it over one shoulder, you look like Grandma and Aunt Annie.

Rather choose longer scarves that can be wrapped around your neck several times, or wrapped around both shoulders. Opt for more modern versions made from cotton or lightweight knits and select it in different vibrant colours. Be selective with prints though as certain prints like paisley and equestrian prints can make you look older, while floral and geometric prints can create a more youthful image.

A modern way to add a scarf to your outfit, is not to wear it yourself, button attach it to the handle of your handbag, wear it rolled up as a handbag, or wrap it loosely around your waist as a belt if you want to add focus to your waist.

Clinging to the Past Trends

A style that looked good on you many years ago does not necessarily still look good on you now. If it is outdated, it will add many years to your image and people will know that the look you are wearing probably looked good on you many years ago. These outfits include mock turtlenecks, nude pantyhose and twinset pants or skirts.

Rather wear the modern versions of old favorites, such as flat shoes instead of mules and regular turtleneck shirts instead of mock turtleneck shirts. Opaque or textured tights should replace nude hose. Wear twinsets as separate pieces.

Same Look, All the Time

Do not get stuck in a rut. When you always look the same by wearing the same style of clothes, same accessories, the same shoes and use the same handbag, you will inevitably add years to your look. It is an easy mistake to make to think a look suits you and then never altering it.

If you are afraid of change and of what the effect will be, alter your look with little changes at a time. Change your handbag when going to different occasions. Use a clutch bag for a cocktail or formal dinner and leave the heavy duty all in one bag for the shops and use a more professional bag for the office. Start by just using a different bag each for summer and for winter. Experiment with accessories such as jewellery and belts.

A small subtle changes every day will create a more vibrant and youthful image.

Under Accessorizing

Never underestimate the power and effect of accessories. An outfit without it is not complete and will make you look dull and older than your true age.

Not only do accessories complete your outfit, wearing the correct accessories can liven up your outfit and shed many years from your image.

Accessories include wearing the correct shoes with your outfit, jewellery, handbags, belts and even hats.

Playing around with these items and experimenting with different combinations will remind you that fashions are constantly changing and can be a lot of fun.

Mix colours and textures of jewellery to suit your outfit, and choose from an array of earrings from hoops to chandeliers to add emphasis to your outfit.

Wear different clips and pins in your hair, not the functional kind, but the decorative ones. Add hair extensions and add-ons in different lengths and colors to your hair to add volume and depth.

Mom and Dad Slacks

These pants come from the era when smart-casual pants were not available in many different styles, when women first started entering the work place and left the traditional role of housewife and mom. These pants are typically the high waist pants with pleated fronts.

These pants have the tendency to accentuate your problem areas, instead of hiding it.

Rather wear pants with a flat front and that are mid-rise, with a straight or bootleg cut. It will make you look younger with the added benefit of making you look slimmer as the widening towards the bottom of the pants will balance out your hips and bust.

Workout Clothes When You're Not Working Out

This is a very simple rule. If you are not working out, there is no need to wear workout clothes. Gym clothes and trainer tracksuits and shoes are made for just that: to use in the gym and to train in.

If you need to wear the oversized top and stretch pant look, wear stretch denims combined with longer knit tops, or choose certain name brands whose gym clothes styles are as modern as casual clothes.

And avoid white sneakers in any style. Choose sneakers in different colors to suit your outfit, whether it is with casual or workout clothes.

Certain Pastels

Pastels may be sweet and cute, but wearing it incorrectly can make you end up like looking like candyfloss or Little Miss Muffet.

Rather opt for jewel tones which are more flattering to all complexions, ages and hair colors.

You can still wear pastels, but wear it selectively. Rather wear more subtle pastels and combine it with neutral colors, such as white or grey for a fresh and young look.

Matching Jewellery Sets

Avoid wearing jewellery as a matching set of earrings, bracelet and necklace, especially if has a motif, such as hearts or flowers.

Mix and match different pieces from different sets. Choose one jewellery item as a focal point and add other jewellery pieces that complement the focus pieces, instead of matching it or competing with it.

Another modern trend is to mix different precious metals and colors such as gold and silver together and wearing them together as the same type of jewellery piece, like wearing silver and gold necklace as pairs or stacked as bangles.

Over Accessorising

It is necessary to wear jewellery and/or other accessories to complete your outfit, but when you go overboard with your accessories, you may end up looking like a Christmas tree adorned with all that sparkles. This style can add more years to your image

Elegance is the most important factor when accessorising and overdoing it strips you of that elegance. Use accessories tactfully to accentuate positive characteristics. Wear shimmering items combined with more subtle clothing pieces to balance the outfit, or opt for neutral clothing with a finishing of subtle shimmery effects.

When it comes to shiny details such as sequins, the less of it in your outfit, the more sophisticated will your outfit look.

Wide Legged Cropped Pants

Wearing these flared pants will almost definitely make your legs look short and thick and add years to your look, especially when the length of the pants is halfway between your knee and ankle.

For a more modern and youth creating style, opt for Capri pants, or cropped pants of full length. A flattering style for most women is when the length of the pants is five inches above the ankle.

Always consider your body type and wear the pants to create length and balance your upper body. Avoid the cargo style cropped pants with pockets as side detail to avoid added width at your waist and bottom.

Wearing Clothes Too Young for Your Age

Even though we all want to look younger than we are and clothes are a great way to achieve this goal, it is not a good idea to choose clothes that are meant to be in your kids' closets. When you try too hard to look young and hip, it will in fact make you look older.

Most international brands have mature versions of the younger trends. Instead of wearing a miniskirt, rather opt for a mid-length version that stops a few inches above your knee, or choose knit tights or opaque's with a tunic top instead of tight fitting leggings. The test for an age appropriate item of clothing is to see if it fits in with the rest of your clothes in your wardrobe. If an item is not in the department you usually shop in, it is not age appropriate. You should never go to the teenager department to buy an item for yourself if you are not a teenager.

Being Too Safe

Signature look should never be confused with getting stuck in a rut and choosing the too safe options.

You can still wear your signature items, but make it more interesting by choosing interesting cuts and details on basic items. Try a flare out A-line shirt and even perhaps a modern belt with it, instead of a plain white button-up shirt, to pair with a tan or black pants. Or choose the safe shirt and pants, but wear it with a bold coloured jacket. Wear metallic strappy sandals or pumps instead of your safe brown shoes or those thick rubber soles and square toes.

Wedge heeled shoes are very trendy and more comfortable than stiletto's and goes with most outfits.

Retro Styles Worn in Old Fashioned Ways

When wearing styles that made a comeback from previous years, do not wear it exactly the same way as you did the first time it made fashion highlights. This is to avoid making you look as if you got stuck in that era. It is then easy for you to give away your true age.

Revive and refresh your classics by pairing them differently with more modern pieces of clothing. Your secretary shirt will look more youthful when worn with a jean and wedge heeled shoes. Or add a cashmere scarf paired with your calf length skirt and long sleeved t-shirt that is tucked in. Or wear different length of chains and pearls with it.

Underperforming Underwear

Underwear, top and bottom, should fit correctly and provide the support required from it. The back of a bra, for instance, should fit under your shoulder blades and not between or above it. When a bra does that, it will drag your bust down proportionally. Breasts that drag downward have never been a sign of youth.

Visible panty lines are a big problem for many women and style experts. If it does not fit properly, it will create lumps and bulges in your rear.

Have yourself measured by a specialist of clothing and image to avoid wearing underwear that creates muffin top hips and stomachs and those that create unsightly bulges.

Another good option to consider is shape. Wear it to create control in problem areas and makes your clothes look smoother, shedding many years from your image.

Box Cuts

Not having a young body, is no reason to wear formless clothing. As you age, it becomes more and more important for you to wear clothes that fit properly.

Wear well-fitted clothes and styled clothing pieces that can accentuate certain areas and good points and to conceal negative parts.

If your body has lost form due to age, then it can be corrected by wearing clothes that create form.

Chapter 3: 7 Personal Steps to Follow for Looking Younger

Find out why you want to be "adorable"

There are many reasons people want to feel special, or adorable and adorable can mean different things to different people.

It can mean you want to feel special, or want to look good, or perhaps you want to get that special attention from somebody.

To be adorable, is not just a physical aspect, like looking good, it is an attitude and a personality trait. It is an overall picture of yourself and what you portray to the world.

Adorable not only applies to girls. Boys can also be adorable and the same steps for being adorable and respected apply to both girls and boys.

Have an image in your mind of what you want to look like

First of all you need to decide what you perceive adorable to be. Then only can you form an image of yourself and what image you want to have.

Decide what image you want to have, such as an innocent look, or a more edgy and modern look. It then becomes easier to find inspiration by looking through magazines, browsing the internet or speaking to image consultant.

When you know what goal you are working towards, it becomes easier to find the tools and tricks to achieve that goal and to create the look you want to achieve.

Improve your hygiene

Looking after yourself and your personal hygiene is always the first step to looking good. If you are not serious about looking after yourself, no one else will take you seriously.

Keeping your body and your hair clean and neat, will create a positive image with people you interact with.

You do not need to have perfect teeth to keep them clean and sparkly and nothing makes a smile look better than having pearly whites! Chew breath mints between brushing your teeth.

Bath or shower at least once a day and make sure that there are no traces of residue left of cream or perfume from the previous day. Rinse properly to avoid a new build-up of soap and suds.

Moisturise your skin daily to keep it soft and supple and prevent premature aging.

In certain circumstances it is not necessary to wash your hair every day. Washing hair too much can over stimulate oil glands and make your hair appear oilier. Wash hair every second day to allow the natural oils of your hair to distribute through your hair and nourish it naturally. It is necessary to wash your hair daily if you are prone to oily hair especially if it appears oily easily.

Keep finger nails clean and clipped to a good length. Men should have short, neatly clipped nails and women can have longer nails, as long as it is well-groomed. Too long nails can look neglected and even make you look older that you are. Do not bite your nails. Get appropriate help if you are a nail biter, or stick fake manicured nail tips on your nails.

Layer your fragrances and creams of the same brand to create a long lasting fragrant scent throughout the whole day.

Adopt good hygiene routines such as washing your hands after you used the bathroom and after handling pets.

Feel special!

Feeling special will boost your self-esteem and when you feel special, you will necessarily carry an image of looking special.

Treat yourself to a sauna treatment or massage. Have your hair done by a professional stylist. These small things can not only make you feel more positive and relaxed, it will shed years off your image.

If you do not have the means for such treats, start by doing the basics. Pamper yourself with a facial mask at home, or a luxurious homemade facial scrub made from honey and oats.

An at home pedicure for your feet will relieve you of stress that has built up and relax your senses when combined with some aromatherapy oils.

If you are a woman that does not usually wear make-up, try wearing a little bit of make-up each day. Start by applying some concealing makeup and foundation and then add lipstick and even some mascara if you are feeling brave.

It is amazing what difference just a little make-up can do when you apply it correctly. Make-up has the power to not only hide problems, but can also accentuate your best facial features. Choose a focal point on your face and work around that.

To achieve the full effect of make-up, be aware of certain small details. Make-up looks better on a clear and clean face that has been moisturised. Always keep your lips soft and supple before applying lipstick and apply foundation to your face before applying make-up.

You should exercise regularly to keep your blood circulation optimal and to keep your heart performance at a healthy level. Exercising regularly will put a natural blush on your cheeks.

Improve your attitude

You can be the prettiest and skinniest person on earth, but if you have a bad attitude, unfortunately it will get you nowhere when your goal is to be adorable and noticed. By improving your attitude, your interactions and responses from other people will also improve.

The best way to immediately improve your attitude is to smile. A warm and honest smile is an invitation to people to communicate with you. Being unfriendly and showing negative emotions are sure ways of driving people away from you.

Be friendly and nice towards other people. Good manners and decency doesn't cost a cent, but it means millions to the people around you. Avoid being overly friendly and don't try to be someone you are not just to impress other people. It is difficult to keep up such a charade.

Be yourself, each person is unique. Be loyal and trustworthy and be considerate. Without these traits, it will be easier to distance people from you, than to attract people. Don't be afraid to make new friends and take the first step. Do not be dependent on other people to live your live. You are in control of your own destiny.

Accessorize

Do not always accept certain things for what they seem to be. Make effort to improve your image by using the correct accessories, including jewellery, shoes, scarves and bags. You have no reason to just accept your straight upper body if you can create the illusion of a trim waist by adding a belt to your outfit.

Accessories are a great way to achieve a certain look. Wear fine jewellery with precious or semi-precious stones for a more romantic look, or beads and stacked bangles for a more casual look. Wear bows, clips and hair bands for a trendy look.

Men do not have to stand back when it comes to accessorising. Jewellery and other accessories for men have become very modern and updated and more acceptable to wear. It is not necessary for men to only be seen wearing a wedding ring. Bracelets and arm bands are very fashionable and come in trendy styles such as leather straps or chains.

Bandanas and beanies are always popular choices for men to wear to achieve a more edgy and youthful look. It is young and vibrant and many celebrity men are seen regularly sporting the beanie look.

Certain accessories are seasonal, so it is good to wear it for a trendy and modern look, but do not wear outdated seasonal styles. Always have a few classic pieces in your accessory collection and even look for certain seasonal styles that can be worn as classic styles. Mix seasonal styles and classic styles and try to find your own individual style that you feel comfortable in.

Stay Kind and Confident

Confidence is one of the best attributes to have. When you are confident, your body language shows you are confident. An important thing about confidence is to be you and stay true to yourself.

Being true to yourself means to accept yourself as you are and not let small things bother you, especially regarding image. No one wants to be around a person who is constantly complaining about their size and weight. Everybody is unique and special and your body type does not determine your personality. Don't allow people to bring you down and tell you otherwise.

Be positive and be kind to other people. Greet people back when they greet you, smile and make eye contact. Help people when help is needed, even if it is something that may seem insignificant, such as help someone cross the street. Help out sometimes at your local animal shelter or volunteer at a soup kitchen.

Above all believe in yourself and be sincere. Remember the Prayer for Serenity by Reinhold Niehbur: "God, grant me the serenity to accept the things I cannot change, the courage to change the things I can and the wisdom to know the difference."

Chapter 4: Using Colors through Make-Up to Enhance Your Look

Learn What Colors Convey

Colors play an important role to send out particular message and can indicate your personality.

- Dark colors like black and blue sends a message of authority

- Pastel colors indicate you are relaxed and friendly. Some pastel colors to wear are mint green and light purple.

- Mixing colors successfully shows you are creative. Wear colors that complement each other like mixing berry colors with red

- Red can have different messages, depending on the nuances you are wearing. Wear burgundy to show sophistication, blue-red to indicate you are assertive and an orange-red to show vibrancy.

- Pink is a good color to wear to show you are openhearted. Pink indicates love and kind-heartedness, compassion and warmth.

- White stands for purity, freshness and a new beginning.

- Yellow gives the impression of warmth and optimism. It symbolises the sun, light and energy and can have the same life giving and healing qualities that the sun has.

- Orange is for energy and all that goes with energy. It is bold, lively and vibrant.

Cool or warm complexions

In the next section, you will learn that each person has a season determined by their skin tone, but before you can determine your season, you first have to know whether you have a cool or warm undertone.

There are different ways in which you can determine your undertone. In this section, two options will be discussed.

The first way is to look at the veins on your forearm while you are in natural light. If your forearm looks pink and the veins blue, then you have a cool undertone. With a warm undertone, your forearm will have a yellow tone and the veins will look greener.

A second way to determine your undertone, is to look in a mirror with a silver piece of paper held next to your face, and after that holds a gold piece of paper next to your face. If you note a more bluish color, your undertone is cool, and a warm undertone will display a more yellow undertone.

Warm undertones are usually found at people who have a golden skin color or skin with a yellowish colouring, while people with cool undertones tend to have red cheeks or a slight ruddiness.

Determine Your Season

Each person has a season that is determined according to your skin tone and hair color. Knowing your season is essential when choosing make up colors and colors of clothing.

Now that you know if you have a cool or warm undertone, you can determine your season.

Winter and summer both have a cool undertone.
- Winter skin tones usually have the cool skin tone, but with dark hair. They have a big contrast between hair and eye color, and skin tone. If you are a winter skin tone, don't wear neutral and earthy colored clothes; rather wear rich colors such as red and blue which will flatter your skin tone and style.

- Summer skin tone people will have light hair and skin with the cool undertone. With their light skin tones, summer people look best in pastel colored clothes and clothes with neutral tones. Bright colors will make your already light complexion look paler.

Spring and autumn have warm undertones.

- Spring, along with the warm undertone, you also have light hair, such as blond, light brown and red hair. Wear colors that are pale and clear. You can also wear bright colours to enhance your skin tone. Do not wear dark colored clothes as it will make you look paler.

- Autumn people have a darker skin tone darker hair: red, brown and black. They can wear a wide variety of colors, but should avoid pastels and bright colors.

Tips and warnings

Do not be afraid to mix colours. Your favorite color and the color that looks best on you may sometimes differ. Mix the colors as it will enhance not just your image, but also your mood. It is after all you that is wearing the clothes and the best trait for a good image, is self-confidence. In a situation where the colors differ, wear the color that suits your skin tone near your face; wear the favourite color as an accessory, such as a handbag.

If you like a color, but it does not suit you, try the color in a different hue, such as wearing turquoise instead of jade. Also balance out colors when you are wearing bold items or colors. Use more subtle make up colors to balance the bold colors.

When choosing colors to wear, be aware that colors also have an individual under tone and that the color itself is no indication whether it is warm or cool. A color may appear to be warm, such as red, but in fact it has a blue undertone, making it a cool color.

Experiment with colors. Do not wear the same color for your whole outfit, even though the color suits you. Mix and match other colors that complement that color and enhance it.

Assess Your Choices

The combination of your hair color can determine which clothes and colors to wear. Assess your combination and make your choice from there.

Blond hair

- When you have blue eyes with blond hair, blue, blue-greens, light greens and turquoise are flattering colors to wear.

- If you have blond hair and green eyes clothes and make up in shades of green, orange and blue enhance your complexion very good.

- Hazel and brown eyes with blond hair, is a good combination to wear purples, pinks, reds, oranges and browns.

- A person with blond hair and grey eyes can wear any colour as your grey eyes will reflect any color. The only color to avoid is light yellow.

Brown hair

- People with brown hair and blue eyes should wear clothes and make up in shades of red, orange, pink and yellow.

- When you have green eyes and brown hair, you can also wear reds, pinks, oranges and yellow, but you can also add green to your pallet.

- People with hazel and brown eyes and brown hair should go for colors in earth and dark tones. Blue also suits your complexion.

- For people with brown hair and grey eyes, you will look good in black and greys. To break the monotony of grey and black, add hues of blue and purple to create an effective impression.

Red hair

- Combined with blue or grey eyes, a person with red hair should wear colors of purple, green and light orange and combine it with black

- People with red hair and with green or hazel eyes, looks most flattering when wearing hues of green (dark or light), purple and earthy colours of red.

Dark hair

People with dark hair, regardless of their eye color, can wear any color combination. Be aware to not only wear neutral colors such as black and brown, but weave in color to add depth and personality to your image.

Chapter 5: Picking the Right Outfit

Picking an outfit for a specific occasion with limited time may seem overwhelming sometimes, but it is possible to select the perfect outfit for any occasion if you work according to a plan.

Assess the occasion

First you need to determine where you are going and what the occasion is. The occasion will determine the outfit. You also need to determine what statement you want to make, do you want to stand out from the crowd, or do you want to make a statement, but still blend in with everyone else.

Determine your style

For a classier look, combine khaki pants with a silk top, or any more formal pants with a sophisticated blouse. A smart casual outfit works for most occasions unless otherwise specified. Lace and silk combined with smart casual pants always creates a classier image. Vintage pants are also good options, especially when combined with a more feminine blouse.

For a more casual look, a vintage jean will look good with tank tops. Try a lace trim for a bit more feminine touch.

Key items and finishes

Clothes can be layered for a more interesting look. Wear a cropped top over a vest or a long sleeved shirt, or a shirt over a lace trimmed tank top. A short skirt worn over a pair of leggings is very modern and creates a young and funky image.

Choose certain key items of clothing and build the rest of your outfit around that item. One statement item is enough and the other items should complement that item, such as a silk blouse worn with more neutral smart casual pants.

Shoes to go with your outfit

Shoes should be chosen to go along with your outfit. For a sophisticated look you can wear heeled sandals or open toed shoes with heels. Heels create length and a slimmer image. Wear sneakers with jeans for a more casual or sporty look. Wear sandals or pumps with a casual pants and a pretty top for a smart casual look.

Applying makeup

Apply makeup after you are dressed to avoid smears on your clothes. Apply makeup according to the under tone and season of your skin tone and hair. Apply the colors to balance out the colors of your clothing. Wear bolder colors of makeup with subtle colored clothing and more neutral makeup and foundation when you are wearing a statement item of clothing.

Accessories

Accessories can change the whole image of your outfit. Wear subtle earrings to enhance a classy outfit and create sophistication. Wear belts to emphasise your waist with a stylish blouse and choose the correct handbag to create the desired effect.

Wear a blazer or coat with your outfit. It will instantly make you look younger and it works in any season, even summer. A trench coat suits any age. To have one in a neutral color, will fit with every outfit. A classic color such as red will transform any outfit with a splash of color.

Crotchets and knitwear are great ways to hide your age. Not only is it very trendy and can be worn over anything, it also adds extra warmth in cooler days. Wearing a crotchet top or vest over a tank top as outerwear is very sexy and feminine and you can wear it to any occasion, be it to the beach or work.

Doing your hair

Your hair should be done after you are dressed so that your clothes does not undo your hairstyle. It will also help to first assess your image after you are dressed to determine what style to wear your hair in. Certain steps can be done the night before, such as braiding your hair to create waves when you loosen it. Remember to wear accessories in your hair that matches your outfit. Pretty bows and clips will work for a playful image, while more subtle or bejewelled clips and bands are great hair accessories to create more sophistication.

Tips and warnings

The combination of jeans worn with a denim jacket is outdated. Do not discard your favorite items; rather use them in different and more modern ways. Rather wear a cropped jacket or tailored jacket with your jean, or wear the denim jacket with an A-line skirt for a more country styled look.

Pastels heeled shoes can be worn with a vintage skirt for a soft and feminine spring look. Combine it with a neutral colored tank top.

Be unique and be yourself. Create your own signature. Wear clothes that you feel comfortable in and that suit you.

If a certain style is high fashion, it does not mean you are forced to also wear it, especially if it does not suit you. As mentioned previously, if a certain color does not suit you, perhaps consider a different hue of that color.

If the style does not suit your body type, apply the rules for dressing to accentuate your better features and hide your flaws. Wear the blouse that is in fashion, but choose it in a darker color to slim down your upper body, or wear denim, but choose low-rise denim to add volume to your hips if your hips and waist are the same width.

Sharp and contrasting colors creates a younger image, while dull colors looks faded and creates the idea that the item has been washed a few times too many. This may lead people to think that you have had that item for ages.

When you wear an item with geometric designs, wear a plain item with it. Wearing two different items with geometric design may look busy and excessive. Rather pair one item as the key item and then add a plain blouse or pants with it to create balance.

Be bold and experimental and do not let any person or fashion style dictate who you should be.

Chapter 6: Coordinating Your Outfit

- Pick out the favorite top

- Selecting another that matches your chosen color

- Jeans or pants that matches your chosen color

- Try different accessories with your chosen outfit

Are you still unsure of how to coordinate your outfit? It is normal, because it is human nature to want to feel your best and to feel your best; you have to look your best. At least you want to be comfortable and self-confident when you face the world. Follow these basic steps and it will be a breeze to coordinate the perfect outfit.

First, you need to pick your favourite top or blouse. Choose that you feel good in and that compliments your personality, your body shape and your season. Also, decide whether you want to layer your shirts or wear it on its own.

If you are planning to layer your clothing and you have chosen a multi-colored shirt as an undershirt, decide which of those colors is your favorite. That color will be handled as the primary colour.

Choose your next shirt according to the primary color. Wear this shirt over the first one, or under it. Layering your clothes is very modern and in fashion. Choose pieces that complement each other to create a younger image.

When you have your shirts chosen and coordinated, it is time to select your pants or skirt. If your shirt has patterns or multiple colours on it, choose a bottom that is single colored. To keep to the layering effect, women can wear a pair of tights with a miniskirt or dress. Choose a funky pair of opaque's for a vibrant look, lace for a more romantic look or plain for a classic style.

Choose your shoes according to your outfit. Boots works wonderful with tights and layered shirts, if you are a woman. Wearing pumps with a denim or skirt will create a soft and delicate image. Your shoes should improve the balance created by your clothes. Do not wear flat shoes if you want to add length to your outfit.

Men should choose their shoes according to the style of the outfit. Wear sneakers for a sporty and casual look. Boots will work for a more rugged look. Dress shoes should go with a suit for a more formal look. Men's' shoes have become more fashionable over the years and the variety are great. There is no need for men to stand back when it comes to fashion!

The last part is the fun part: accessorise! Accessories are important not only to complete your outfit, but also to emphasise your good features and draw attention away from your not so good features. Choose accessories that match the color and style of your outfit. Experiment with your accessories, wear different pieces in different complementing colors.

Tips and warnings

Do research on the latest fashions; what should be worn together and what to avoid. To avoid spending unnecessary money on magazines, swap magazines between you and your friends, or watch the fashion programs on satellite television.

The most important thing to remember when coordinating your outfit is color. Make color the center point. Color is used to balance out body shapes, it is used to complement your skin tone and season and it can be used to indicate your personality. Color can transform a whole outfit from negative to positive by just making a few simple changes.

If you are wearing a very simple outfit, add a few key points like accessories to liven up the outfit. Add colorful accessories to brighten up your image. Be creative with accessories. Wear multi-colored bangles or layer your necklaces. Hair accessories are very trendy and come in various designs and colors.

Both black and white are versatile colors and you can wear it with any other color. The key is style to add color, do not wear just black or just white, even if you just add colored accessories.

Be creative, be original, and wear your outfit with confidence. Round off your outfit with a smile.

Chapter 7: Accessorise Your Outfit

When choosing accessories, you have to bear in mind the overall image of your outfit and what you want to achieve with your outfit and to which occasion you are wearing your outfit. Accessories should be an extension of not only your outfit, but of your personality.

Jewellery

Jewellery is the most important accessory. Jewellery is a personal choice and unique to your personality. You should therefore choose your jewellery selectively and wisely.

Select your focal point item and select the other items to match or complement the focus item. Usually your necklace is your focus point, but it is not the rule. The other option for a focus item, are earrings. Choose your other jewellery according to one of these.

Earrings place emphasis on your face and neck and can reflect light and color to your face. Choose long earrings or drop earrings if you have a round face and hoops for an oval face.

The same applies for necklaces. Choose a long necklace to elongate a short neck and a chunkier or short necklace for a long neck. Wear a chocker with a long neck to make it appear shorter.

Your watch should be a good quality watch and made of neutral colors to suit all your clothing. Watches with leather or gold straps are good choices that suit most clothing.

If you want to add more emphasis to your arms, wear bracelets. Experiment with bracelets. There are more styles than just regular bangles. Go for a more sophisticated look with a cuffed style bracelet, or more feminine with a delicate chain or charm bracelet. Try wrapping a leather strap around your wrist for a tribal look.

You should also distinguish your jewellery between daywear and eveningwear. Choose casual jewellery made of beads, seeds, wood and less jewels on more casual outfit. Flashy items with many jewels should be worn to formal occasions and with evening wear.

Head accessories

Hair accessories have survived throughout the ages. New styles have come on board and old favorites are constantly redesigned to suit the latest fashions.

It is very important to wear hair accessories that complement your outfit. If you are portraying a certain style, choose accessories also in that style. With the wide variety of hair accessories available, there will most certainly be an item on the list that will suit your outfit.

The most popular hair accessories are pins and clips. Clips come in all shapes and sizes, from the big jaw clip, to tiny jaw clips and alligator clips. Depending on the length of your hair, hair clips can be used to hold hair together and out of your way, or you can use it to make hairstyles.

The headband is also a favorite. They are available in hard or soft options. The hard headband usually only goes from ear to ear over your head, while the soft material bands wraps around your head. Bands should fit comfortably. If it hurts you, it is too small and you should get a bigger one.

Scarves can be worn as a head accessory and is very versatile. It can be worn as bandannas, rolled up and wrapped around your head as a headband, or you can wear it to cover your head and hair. This is very handy when you go out, but need to keep your style in place.

Another option for both men and women, are hats. Hats are coming back in style in various designs. You get beanies, baseball caps, golf caps and cowboy hats, to name only a few. Hats with wide rims and caps are good to provide extra protection against the sun. Woollen beanies and fur lined trapper hats are invaluable during winter months to provide warmth. Hats are great accessories to theme parties and events to round off your intended theme.

Tiaras are crown like accessories and worn at special occasions. Tiaras should be worn with care to avoid looking like a princess from a fairy tale. Wear tiaras to your wedding or to fancy dress parties.

Belts

Belts can be a very important part of your outfit. Belts are accessories, and should not be worn as necessities. Belts are there to emphasise a lean waist, or create the illusion of a slim waist if you have a straight body type.

If you are not sure or confident on how to wear a belt, here are a few guidelines:

Determine where to wear your belt, where does it suit you the best. It can be at your waist, just above your waist or around your hips.

Next you should consider the width of the belt. Wear a wide belt if you have a long waist and upper body. A person with a short waist should rather wear a skinny belt.

Belts look good when worn over a dress or shirt. Coordinate the colour of the belt to blend in with your clothes. Wear a black belt to create contrast with any color for a dramatic effect, or a silver belt for a more romantic look.

The material which the belt is made of can also play a role in your confidence. Elastic belts are very flexible and comfortable as it adjusts to your body. If a belt becomes uncomfortable, you will be more aware of it and will draw more attention to it as you constantly try to adjust your belt.

Add an extra jacket or shirt for a layered effect, exposing the belt only partially. It creates a unique subtle emphasis on the belt, but also covers the rest of your middle, hiding the less perfect areas.

Getting used to wearing a belt takes a little time. Get to know yourself and your style. When you found your style, you will be able to wear a belt with confidence.

Scarves

Scarves are fun accessories to wear and can be worn throughout the year, not only in winter time. No one can argue about the extra warmth scarves provide during winter. There are many ways how to fashionably wear scarves to complete an outfit.

For an elegant look, wear a scarf in the same color as your outfit when wearing a neutral color. Add one or two items of a different hue to break the monotony of one color. Mix different textures to give even more dimension to your outfit. You can for instance wear a woollen scarf with a woven top

A scarf is worn around your neck, which almost immediately will draw attention to your face. For this reason you need to wear a color that suits your skin tone and season.

You can make a scarf your only accessory and focus point, especially when worn in a contrasting color. Avoid though that scarf does not look as if it is choking you. Drape the scarf loosely around your neck or tie it only once. Take care when wearing a scarf with evening wear as it can easily look unsophisticated. Rather wear a pashmina or sheer scarf draped over your shoulders with evening wear.

A scarf can add color and warmth to a plain outfit. It can make your outfit seem more playful, yet elegant when you drape a shawl or scarf over one shoulder and twisted around your neck.

Don't just stay with plain scarves. Be brave and try printed scarves. The scarf should match the main color in your outfit.

Handbags

It is a very rare sight to see a woman in public without some sort of handbag. This is because handbags are used as transportation items so you can have your most important items with you everywhere you go. It has become a necessity and not always an accessory anymore. Here are some ideas on how to keep it a necessity, but make it look like an accessory.

You can wear a handbag over your shoulder, under your arm, or you can sling it across your body. You will need to adjust the length of the strap to where the handbag should be. The bag must be in proportion to your figure, that is why you need to adjust the strap to place it at the correct proportion to your body.

Wearing a handbag under your arm, or at the elbow, will place emphasise on your upper body. If you have a large bust, wear a small handbag under your arm, or wear your handbag lower down. The same principle will apply with your waist and your lower body. Avoid large handbags at an area where you do not want emphasis, or balance that area out with a small handbag.

Handbags can be any color and do not have to be the same color as your clothes. Be careful, though not to wear a colored handbag that clashes with your clothes. Choose a color that matches another key item of your outfit, or wear a neutral handbag that works with any color.

If the straps of handbag are too short to wear over your shoulder, rather wear it over your arm or in your hand. A handbag should also not conceal your outfit at any time. This means that even when you reach to get something out of your bag, your handbag should still not spoil your shirt or dress. Rather opt for a clutch bag or a smaller handbag if your handbag is overwhelming you.

Sunglasses

Sunglasses are a fashion statement for many people; they will go so far as to insist on wearing only certain designer brands. Regardless what the brand of your sunglasses is, the main function is and should always be to protect your eyes from the harmful rays of the sun.

When choosing a pair of sunglasses, it is important to make sure that the frame suits the shape of your face. A person with an oval face can wear almost any style of sunglasses, while a square face will look softer with round frames. A person with a long face should wear sunglasses with a short frame to shorten the face and a person with a round face type will look good when wearing an angular framed pair of sunglasses.

Sunglasses with prints and colors are fun to wear and you can match it to many outfits. It creates a vintage style. Stay with a classic style if you do not feel comfortable with a too trendy pair, but experiment with the frame of the sunglasses.

Shoes

Shoes are the last part of your outfit and should not only complete your outfit but it should also complement it. It is therefore important that you choose the correct shoes to go with your outfit.

When you purchase shoes, or decide on a pair to wear, always remember the number one rule for shoes: Shoes should fit properly. Never buy or wear a pair of shoes that are too small or big or hurt you in some place, regardless of how pretty they are. If it does not fit properly when you fit them, imagine how your feet will feel at the end of the day. And it tends to spoil even the best outfit if you cannot walk properly.

There are a few points to consider when choosing your shoes:

- What type of outfit are you wearing?

- What is the occasion?

- What is the main color or colors of your outfit?

- Should your shoes help correct an imbalance in your body type?

The type of outfit is determined by the season. If it is winter and you are wearing winter clothes, you cannot wear summer shoes with your outfit. Your shoes should also be winter shoes. If you are wearing a bathing suit, you will also not wear pumps with it, but rather flip-flops. Basic rule: the season of the shoes should match the season of your outfit.

The occasion will also influence your shoe choice. If the occasion asks for casual clothes, then wear casual shoes such as ballet flats and wear pumps for events where you should dress up, such as office work. Wear sneakers when going to the gym or to a sports match or any event that requires a lot of action and physical movements.

The color of your shoes will also be determined by the color of your outfit. You can wear black shoes with basically anything. If you are not certain if the shoes will match the outfit, repeat the color of the shoes somewhere in your outfit. By repeating a color of your outfit with the same color of shoes, you not only match the shoes, you also create an elegant image.

Wear brown shoes with earthy colored clothes and white shoes with light colored clothes or pastels. Golden shoes look good with dark colored or earth toned clothes, while silver shoes work well with blue, purple and red clothes.

Jeans

Jeans have survived throughout the ages. To this day, it is still one of the items that are most bought and worn. It is comfortable, comes in shapes and designs to suit every figure and age and it goes well with everything.

Jeans can be dressed up or down and you can go from one occasion to the next by just changing a few items. You can wear a jean to work with an elegant blouse and a pair of pumps. When at home, substitute the blouse with a sweater and the pumps with ballet flats and you are ready to go shopping!

The only events where jeans are normally not allowed are cocktail parties and black tie events.

Jeans come in various colors with the most famous still being blue and black. Wear dark jeans if you want to create a leaner effect and lighter jeans to balance out a wide upper body. Just the warning again as mentioned in a previous chapter: Please avoid wearing jeans paired with a denim jacket!

How to complement patterns

It is unwise to match too many patterns together as you may end up looking like the circus clown still in need of your red nose. When you choose to wear an item with patterns, it is important to do so wisely.

Always pair patterned items with solid clothing pieces. If your top is patterned, whether it be stripes or floral, match it up by wearing a pants with a solid color. The color does not necessarily need to be repeated by the color in the pattern, but at least make sure that the colors match or complement each other.

Avoid prints with a tiny motif, especially if it reminds you of wallpaper from Biggies Best. It is supposed to be a vintage style, but in fact, it only makes you look older. Rather wear clothing with bold prints.

Work with a colour wheel. Colours next to each other on the colour wheel, creates harmony, while colours opposite each other on the wheel matches by creating a dramatic effect.

If you are weary of wearing patterned clothing, then use wear patterns on your accessories such as shoes, scarves or the frame of your sunglasses. Do not be afraid to experiment and to create your own signature look.

Tips and warnings

Do bargain hunting to get amazing jewellery. Search online at auction sites or other websites selling second hand items. Visit charity shops. Charity shops are not only good for finding bargain priced items; your chances are also good to find a few vintage items. Second hand shops may also be hiding that forgotten treasure.

Make your own jewellery by buying beads, charms, string and straps. Make necklaces, bracelets and earrings from these items. Not only will it save you money, but you will also be guaranteed of a unique and one of a kind piece of jewellery. You can also customise the jewellery to suit your various outfits and colors.

Colors that are gaining popularity are shades of yellow, especially mustard. It works well with plain colors such as black and white.

Add bright colors to an outfit with neutral colors. It will instantly create a youthful image to your outfit.

Chapter 8: Accessorising with Jewellery

Accessories ultimately complete your outfit and should complement your outfit. It can turn any outfit from drab to fab; you only need to know how to use the accessories correctly to achieve that effect. Here are a couple of steps and ideas on how you can successfully coordinate your jewellery to your outfit.

Coordinate with your hair color

Your hair color and skin tone has an influence on the clothes and accessories you wear. There really are not any specific rules to follow on which jewellery you may wear and which to avoid.

By now, you have probably determined your season and skin tone. Use this as a guide when choosing jewellery. As a reminder: warm skin tones are spring and autumn and cool skin toned people are categorised as summer or winter.

If your season is spring or autumn, you can wear gold toned colors. The jewellery will make your skin look warm and rich. Spring toned people can choose gold jewellery, corals and bright pink or green. Autumn toned people look good with orange, deep yellow and certain greens. Wearing silver will not look bad, but it will also not enhance your tone, or it will not create enough contrast.

Cool toned people, summer and winters, should wear cooler colors. Summer toned people can wear colors that are clear, blue or with a silver undertone such as violet and also cherry red. Winter toned people will benefit by wearing pastels with a blue tone or colors with an ice undertone. These colors include cool grey, navy blue, blue and pastels hues of pink and blue.

These are just suggestions. At the end of the day, you have to like what you are wearing and you need to feel comfortable. A collection of jewellery organised by the best style fashionista will mean nothing if you do not like what you are wearing or cannot stand a certain color.

Coordinate jewellery with your clothes

The most important rule to remember when coordinating an outfit is to work with color.

It is always about how to wear color and how to use color to accentuate other items. Once you understand this concept, it will be easy to have the same sense of style that celebrities have.

The first thing to consider when choosing jewellery is the fabric of your outfit. A sheer and elegant outfit should be accessorised by sheer jewellery. Junky wooden beads and seeds will not only clash with your outfit, it may even damage it when it snags. Also, take care that the material of all the jewellery matches. If you are wearing a beaded necklace, do not wear a diamond bracelet with it. Rather wear a leather strap or beads. You do not want to end up looking like a kindergarten Christmas tree.

The color of the jewellery should match your outfit. It does not necessarily have to be the same color, but it should complement your outfit. Gold and other warm toned colors go well together, while cool toned jewellery should be worn with jewellery that also has a cool under tone.

Black jewellery is universal and can be worn with most outfits. When in doubt, add another black accessory, such as a belt, to match the jewellery.

Be careful when wearing pearls. Even though pearls are light in color, it does not go well with many colors. Avoid wearing pearls with white clothing, unless it is your wedding day. Wearing pearls with white clothes will create the effect of a dissolved aspirin or may even make you look like a granny. Pearls features at its best when you wear it with red clothing or with gold clothing.

Your clothes should be the focus of your completed outfit. Wear jewellery to complement your outfit and not the other way around. If you are wearing a plain outfit, wear jewellery to make your outfit more interesting. People should notice the full picture, not just the jewellery.

Coordinate jewellery to create an accent

Jewellery can make a big difference to help balance out a specific body shape. It can be applied to your arms, neck, face and upper body.

Wear long or drop earrings to make a short neck look longer, or hoops and studs to make a long neck look shorter. Be careful with hoops though if you do not want to add more volume to your face and cheeks. Rather opt for small rings or sleeper or short drop earrings.

Wearing a necklace correctly can make a difference to you upper body. Wear a long necklace to elongate your upper body or a shorter and chunkier necklace if you have a long upper body.

If you have skinny arms, wear many bangles together, or fine bracelets. Wearing bangles that are too chunky will make you look unbalanced if you are very skinny. For thicker arms, wear chunky bracelets and bangles. A fine bracelet will not be effective and create no accent.

Coordinate the amount of jewellery

You may feel overwhelmed by the idea of coordinating even the amount of jewellery, when in actual fact it is quite simple. With jewellery, the rule applies of "Less is more".

Wear one piece of jewellery as a focus point to create an elegant look. Choose a classic piece, like a diamond pendant necklace and wear a subtle pair of earrings with it. You can also wear rings, but wear no more than two rings to maintain the elegant look.

Combining more than one matching necklaces will create a more casual look. To create a more casual look, wear more necklaces and bangles. This can be done with costume jewellery.

Coordinating your jewellery with other jewellery

Wearing jewellery is a personal choice and you should show your personal style and uniqueness with your jewellery. Fashion rules changed in many ways and a person now has carte blanche to what they want to wear.

Despite free choice, there are still a few rules that apply to create a well informed and organised outfit. The most important is to choose a color and style and stick to it. If you decide on diamonds, do not wear it with other jewellery made of wood or clay.

When wearing more than one necklace, wear two necklaces that are similar. Do not wear a beaded necklace along with costume jewellery chains. Beads can be worn together with glass jewellery.

If you decide on an antique style, wear only antique pieces that match and not modern or bohemian type or other types of styles. You can wear shiny jewellery with other jewellery, but be careful of going too shiny so as not look like bling draped rap artist.

Arm accessories can be combined successfully too. You can wear a bracelet with your watch, but make sure that the colors of each match each other.

Rings should also be in the chosen style. Your wedding rings, however, are exempted from this rule and other rings and jewellery do not need to be a match to your wedding rings.

Chapter 9: Choose the Right Jewellery for Your Skin Tone and Face Shape

By now you should have already determined your skin tone and the shape of your face. By knowing this, it may save you a lot of frustration when you are shopping for jewellery or trying to coordinate an outfit.

Determine your skin tone

As a reminder of determining your skin tone, you can do the vein test. Look at the inside of your arm in natural light. If your veins appear greenish, you have a warm undertone and if it is a shade of blue, your skin tone is cool. These people normally have dark or tan skin color. If you have a warm skin tone, you should notice a yellow or golden apricot undertone in your skin, while people with a cool skin tone should have a pink or rose undertone in their skin. People with a warm skin tone usually have red hair, or a hair color with a red under tone in, such as strawberry blond, orange and reddish brown. They also normally have a lighter skin.

Choosing a precious metal to wear

You need to know which metal suits you best and work most effectively with your skin tone. After you have determined your metal, you need to choose which gem and color goes best with the metal and your skin tone.

Cool skin tone people can wear silver, white gold and platinum jewellery. Gems to choose from are pearls and diamonds. Choose precious stones that are pink, purple or red. Basically any stone with a blue undertone.

People with warm skin tones should wear jewellery with a yellow undertone, such as gold, copper and brass. They can also wear pewter. They can add gems such as golden toned pearls and coral. Wearing gems such as sapphire, turquoise, orange and brown will also complement a warm skin tone.

Shape of your face

There are four basic shapes for faces: oval, round, heart and rectangular. If you do not know the shape of your face, stand in front of a mirror and pull your hair back and secure with an elastic band. Trace your face with a whiteboard marker. You will be able to notice a specific prominent shape when you look in the mirror.

A round face is characterised by being equally long as it is wide. Your face is soft and stays youthful longer. It ages gracefully. Wear jewellery that has vertical lines and is angled. It will help to make your face look a longer.

When you have an oval face, your face is slightly longer than the width and sometimes displays sharp facial features. Oval faces can also be soft and curved. People with oval faces can wear most jewellery shapes and styles. It is the most versatile face shape to have.

When your face is rectangular, your face is clearly longer than it is wide. When you measure your face in 2 halves, you will find that the length from your forehead to your cheekbone is relatively the same as the length from your cheek bone to your chin. A person with a rectangular face should wear jewellery to create an effect that widens your face. Choose hoops or big drop earrings.

The fourth face shape is a heart shaped face. This face shape is wide at your eyebrows, but narrow at your chin. To balance out this shape, you should wear jewellery that creates width at your chin. Teardrop earrings or drop earrings with a feature towards your chin should suffice.

While coordinating jewellery with your face shape, also consider the length of your neck. The basic rule is that long earring elongates your neck and hoop earrings helps to shorten your neck.

Tips for buying jewellery

To save time, shop at a store where jewellery is organized according to the metal and the color. Most big department stores already groups different metals together and they also add complementary colored jewellery and gems to the groups.

To prevent tarnish on jewellery, you can cover it with a thin layer of clear nail varnish. This tip is very useful when you are not wearing real gold or silver. This saves you money and will lengthen the lifespan of your costume jewellery. Also keep your jewellery away from water to avoid rust.

Wear jewellery that you are comfortable with and makes you feel special and comfortable. Wear something that is unique to you and shows your personal style. You should make the jewellery look good, not the other way around.

One last word of warning: make sure your jewellery does not cause an allergic reaction to your skin. Many people have skin that is sensitive, even to certain metal types. Take note of allergic reaction and try alternatives for that metal type.

Chapter 10: Accessorise a Simple Wardrobe

You do not need a warehouse full of clothes to look gorgeous every day. All you need is the right clothing, the right accessories and the creativity to combine these two elements. With a few key items in your wardrobe you can create an outfit for every day of the week.

So how do you achieve this minimalist wardrobe, you may ask. It is actually very easy once you understand and master the basic principles.

Do your research

Research comes in all forms and formats. The most practical way is to observe other people. You may sit on a bench one day and a person with an interesting outfit or idea may walk past you igniting an idea in your head that you never thought about. It is also a good way to see what styles are popular currently.

If you know your body type and are able to recognise it in other people, you can see how they dress to look good or what to avoid. Observe what jewellery they wear and how they wear it. What materials they match and with what clothes do they wear it.

Look through magazines to get ideas, or surf the internet. Compare your own personal style with the information you have acquired and then customise your wardrobe and accessories accordingly. Know what is not flattering and what makes you feel uncomfortable.

Be creative and resourceful

Use the knowledge you have gained and use the accessories you already have and be creative with it. To be creative means that you must be open for suggestions and improvisation. Use a necklace that you do not wear anymore, or that that does not suit you, as a bracelet on your arm. Wrap it several times around your wrist to create a look of several bangles.

Use a scarf as a belt or wear some of your outdated clothes in a modern way. If you had a skirt and jacket set you wore when you first started working, wear the skirt with a more modern shirt and shoes and add a belt to add emphasis to your waist. Wear layers of necklaces in different lengths for a more dramatic look. The jacket can be worn with jeans or another pants for a smart casual look. Add some interesting earrings, a matching necklace as focus item and a pair of pumps and you are ready to stun the office.

You do not need to spend a lot of money to get the look you want. You will be surprised at what you can achieve with a little imagination.

Make your own individual style

You are unique with your own personality and your own preferences. There are no rules forcing you to wear certain accessories in specific ways. There are only guidelines and suggestions. It is therefore important that you realise that you have to personalise your own individual style.

If you see a model on the runway wearing a necklace that is high fashion and you know that necklace will never suit you; customise it. Opt for a different color or one made of a different material, such as glass instead of beads.

Take a simple top and work beads onto it. There are handheld craft machines available in craft shops that can attach beads, pins and other pretty buttons unto your clothes. Attach these gems and buttons along the stitching of the pockets on your jeans; make a pattern on your handbag or a unique motif on your shirt. It does not have to be overwhelming, just a subtle change, but something that will leave a lasting impression.

The main idea is that you feel comfortable and self-assured. Your smile and self-confidence is always your best accessory.

Go wild with make-up

Apply the color techniques which you have already learned about your skin tone, season, hair color and eye color. Use this knowledge to apply your make up tastefully. To go wild with your make-up does not mean to go overboard.

Add color to your eyes to accentuate your eye color, eye liner to form your eyes, mascara to define your lashes and a good lipstick for kissable lips. Experiment with different colors until you find the perfect combination to transform your canvas to an oil painting.

Try these tips to make your make up more effective:

- Add a bit of lipstick to your cheeks for color.

- Use lip gloss for shine on lips and to make your lipstick stay on longer

- Get rid of old skin on your lips by brushing your lips very gently with an old soft toothbrush and petroleum jelly

- Add interesting jewels and glitter at your eyes

- Add bronzer to your foundation to give your face a healthy glow

- Use white gel eyeliner to make dull eyes look brighter

- Use concealing cover stick to lighten dark circles under your eyes

- Add a bit of green eye shadow to reduce red skin or eyes

- Add sterile tear eye drops to your eyes regularly to hydrate your eyes. This will avoid it from drying out and cause red and irritated eyes.

- Line your eyes only two thirds on the lower lids if you have small eyes and want to make it appear bigger

- Wear eyebrow liner and shape your eyebrows and frame your face

- Take care of your teeth. Any lipstick looks its best when paired with sparkling white teeth.

Be confident with a bold style

There are many ways to make a stylish statement. By just adding color or accessories, you can make a big difference to your outfit. Many of these items are probably already in your house; you might just be not aware of the difference it can make.

Add a colorful jacket to your outfit and a pair of modern, yet comfortable shoes. Then add a few pieces of jewellery that complement your outfit. Remember to choose only one bold item and plan the rest of your accessories around that item. Too many bold items in one outfit will confuse people to what your style should be.

If your statement piece is a pair of long earrings, do not hide it behind your hair. Wear your hair up or away from your ears. Wear a simple necklace and try to keep your neckline open otherwise. Wearing a polo neck shirt or woollen jersey with a thick collar will hide your earrings.

If you are wearing a bold necklace, leave the attention with the necklace. Do not divert attention away by wearing a bold belt. Your earrings should also be less prominent.

Wear fine bracelets with short sleeved shirts. A three quarter sleeve is the best option to draw attention to your bracelet. Cuffed style bangles and large bangles can be worn over long sleeves if the sleeves does not have a motive, otherwise the bangles will get lost in the motive. Bangles can be pair with bold earrings, yet not too bold if the bangles are your statement piece.

Bohemian styles can mix patterns, multiple statement pieces and bold colors. If you are not planning on a bohemian style, wear simple colors and classic clothes and add a bold statement jewellery piece for a dramatic look.

And again, wear it with confidence. Fashion is a relative concept and there are no wrongs or rights. Wearing your outfit with confidence is the best accessory and fashion tip.

Chapter 11: No Need for You to Spend a Lot of Money to Look Young

Wearing the perfect clothes to make you look young does not have to cost you a fortune. There are many tricks of the trade to help you build up a wardrobe and accessories to suit your needs. All you need to do is follow a few basic guidelines to look like a million dollars without you having to take out a personal loan.

Determine your style

Determining your style is not so hard. All you have to do is look at the clothes in your closet and what key pieces you always wear in which you feel comfortable. It is usually those few items that put a bounce in your step when you wear it.

To build your wardrobe around your personal style, you need to choose the items that are spectacular to you. You will recognise those items as the ones that make you look in a mirror and tell yourself: "Wow, you are one gorgeous person!"

Then get rid of the rest. How do you know it is time to get rid of certain items? These items are usually the ones that you have not worn in the last season. They are also the items that you keep in your closet that are probably too small and you want to keep them for when you lose weight.

Sounds familiar? I thought so. Clothes should always fit properly. If a piece of clothing does not flatter you, it fits too tight or hangs like a bag on you, get rid of it. It is not part of your style anymore. Whether your personal style is classic, romantic, modern, bohemian, or whichever suits you, if the item does not shout "gorgeous" when you wear it, then avoid that item and sponsor it to someone who can make better use of it.

Know the brands you want to target

Each person has his or her own personal preference of clothing brand. If you know your brand preference, it is easier to shop for your clothing. Find out where those brands are available and do your shopping from there.

Branded names are usually more expensive than clothes bought at a department store. Consider to buy your key items from your favorite brand and get complementary items at a more discounted store. The cheaper items are easier to discard of when your style or personal taste changes.

Buy a key piece for every part of your outfit from your favorite brand. The basic pieces to look for are a blouse, pants, a skirt, and a jacket. For accessories you can get a pair of shoes, handbag and jewellery.

Attend discount sales

Classic pieces never go out of style. With this in mind, consider attending an end of season discount sale. If you choose wisely, you will be able to wear that item again the next season and pay a lot less for it than usual.

Look out for relocation sales when shops move from one premises to the other and need to clear their stock to make the relocation easier. The items are still the same brand of the same quality, but at a fraction of the cost.

Another good place to pick up bargains is at charity shops. Many people donate clothes for their own personal reasons. It may be that they have also discovered their own style and is throwing out items that no longer fit in their style. You may be lucky enough to find that those items are in fact your style.

Many stores have regular bargain bins where you can scratch and search for that one unique item that you would have otherwise not be able to afford. You will not be the first or last person to search through a bargain bin. Do not see yourself as stingy; see yourself as a stylish person with a sense for budget and someone who is practical.

Another good place to look for key items, are flea markets. Many people with stalls are either importers of barrels of clothes, which means you can get clothes at discounted prices, or they hand make the clothes they sell, so you will be certain to find a unique item.

Key items to have in your wardrobe

- Dress pants: Have one preferably in black. Black is slimming and can be worn with any color shirt.

- A classic shirt: Every person needs to own at least one classic white shirt. White shirts are available in various styles, so choose a style that flatters your body shape. Make sure it is trendy and not outdated.

- The Any occasion top: This top should be one that makes you feel good and self-confident and you can wear it to any occasion. You should be able to wear it to work, or for a night out, or when going shopping.

- A basic black dress: This classic piece of clothing not only have to be a "little black dress", it can be any length that flatters you and in which you feel comfortable.

- Skirt: Wear a skirt when you need something more feminine than a dress pants. Skirts are available in many styles, from business like to romantic. Skirts are necessary for women to avoid being stuck in a pattern of only wearing pants.

- The Day dress. This item allows you to be more feminine. It is a man's world and women need to put a lot of effort in to succeed. Women tend to forget they are the softer sex and even wear clothes that look like a man. Own at least one dress to wear in daytime to remind you of your femininity.

- Jeans: Jeans have become a fashion statement and with so many styles available these days; it is now possible for every person to own a pair of jeans that makes them look gorgeous.

- Jacket: Jackets are great accessories to round of any outfit. Wear a tailored jacket in the same color as your outfit for an elegant look, or wear one in a funky color for a trendy and modern look.

- Trench coat: A trench coat is classic, but also very trendy. It is available in different lengths and styles to suit any outfit.

- Casual clothes: This can be something alternative to a sweat suit. Jeans may be great, but there are days when you need something a bit more casual to relax in or to snuggle in on winter days. Try something like khaki, cotton or corduroy. It is flexible and comfortable to wear to almost any place.

Classic, yet trendy, according to your body shape

Whether your body shape is diamond, apple or rectangle, the same principles always apply. Once you have determined your body shape, your personal style and the brands you prefer, you will need to get a few pieces of clothing that is classic and will never go out of style.

Choose those items with your body shape in mind to balance out imperfections. That means it will accentuate your good qualities and hide the less good qualities. These items will last you more than one season if you take care of it which is beneficial if you do not want to buy new clothes every season.

Be creative

You will be surprised at what you can achieve with your outfit when you broaden your choices. Use key items and then add your own touch to it. By just making a few small changes, you can transform your whole outfit.

Mix and match items that you do not usually wear together. Wear an item in a different way. Add a different pair of shoes to your outfit or add a hat. Change your hairstyle. If you always wear your hair straightened, leave your hair to air dry and then crunch some styling gel into your hair using your fingers and whole hand, depending on the desired style. Wear your hair with a side path instead of your usual middle path, or have a fringe cut into your hair. It will make a world difference.

Never be afraid to experiment and break the rules until you find your own personal style. You can achieve this by just being more aware of what is happening around you or just by doing stock take on your own closet and dresser and being creative with what you have on hand.

You will never know how good your denim jacket looks with your floral summer dress until you give it a try.

Chapter 12: Find the Perfect Jeans for You

Jeans is a classic item of clothing that never goes out of style. The styles of jeans may change from time to time, but jeans itself never leave the fashion scene. Every person should own at least one pair of jeans and if you don't, now is the time to get a pair for your closet.

Curb your enthusiasm for just a few minutes longer and first read through these important notes on how to select the perfect pair of jeans before you rush to the shops.

By now you should already know what your body shape is and know that it is important to choose clothes according to your body shape. Here are a few tips on what to look for in jeans.

If you have an hourglass figure, choose a wide legged jean to balance your hips and thighs. A mid-rise denim will create width at your waist. Wear a pair of high heeled shoes with your denim to create length and slim down your hips even more.

If you are tall and lean, you probably have a rectangular body. Rectangular body types can wear jeans that have narrow, straight legs. Low rise denim will add width to your hips. Ballet flats will work well for women to avoid giving additional length.

If you have a flat bottom, you can choose a pair of jeans with pockets on your bottom to give more volume. The opposite should be applied when you have a big bottom. Avoid high back pockets so you do not draw unnecessary attention to that area.

For a petite figure, get slim cut jeans, or skinny jeans as they are now called. It will not create unnecessary width to your petite frame. The slim cut legs and middle will accentuate your frame and make you look more feminine. Wear light blue jeans and low rise jeans to make you look curvier. You can also consider jeans in alternative colours, such as gray or brown.

People with a pear shaped body should wear bootleg or flare jeans. This will balance out your hips. Choose a high rise back that will cover your back, but not gape at the front. Avoid jeans that are tapered at the top as you do not want to draw attention to your hips. Buy your jeans in a dark blue or black color to slim you down.

Apple shaped people should wear bootleg jeans with a medium rise back. The bootleg or flare of the jeans will help to balance out your waist and create width at your legs. Your legs are your best feature, so use this to divert attention to your legs.

Tips and rules for wearing denim

- Boot cut jeans with medium rise waist is a style that is flattering to all types of shapes.

- When buying jeans, move around in the fitting room to see how the jeans forms to your body. Make movements as you would do in your daily routines to establish if it will work for you.

- Fit your jeans with shoes you wear regularly. Try them on with ballet flats, sneakers and with pumps to get an overall idea of how it will look.

- Shop where you feel comfortable. If you shop in a store that makes you feel uncomfortable, you will most likely choose the nearest pair of jeans just to get out of the store. You should feel comfortable wearing your jeans, so fit your jeans in a store where you feel comfortable.

- Do not buy the first pair of jeans that you like. Shop around as different designers and brands have different qualities. If the jeans of a certain designer fit well, the jeans of another designer may just fit fantastic.

- When you find good fitted and flattering jeans, buy two of them, one to wear with flat shoes and one to wear with high heels. The reason for this is that you tend to wear out the bottom of your jeans faster when wearing flat shoes and the worn out hem is very unflattering with high heels.

- Throw away old jeans that are faded and worn out. Marks and faded spots tend to draw attention to that part of your body and can make that area appear larger.

- Jeans with high waists should be avoided. It is very unflattering to your waist and your bottom, making it appear very big. Rather find another style that balances out your imperfections and is more flattering.

- Jeans should be appropriate to the occasion. Darker jeans tend to look more formal and are very slimming. Wear an appropriate blouse and accessories to create a formal look. Sparkly tops and accessories work well with dark jeans if you are planning a night out with your friends.

- The basic rule is the darker the jeans, the more formal it is. A crease in the front will give a formal and polished look. Light jeans are for casual wear.

- Wear age appropriate jeans. Wearing jeans that are intended for children will make you look older instead of younger. The rule here: shop in your age section of the store. If the jeans are not in your section, do not buy it for yourself.

- Draw up a budget and stay with it. Do not try on a pair of jeans that you know you cannot afford. You will be too tempted to buy it when you have fixated on it.

- If the hems of your jeans are too long, have it tailored to shorten it. It is unflattering to walk around in new jeans with already worn out hems.

- Just like work trousers, jeans can also be altered. Have your jeans custom made for a perfect fit.

- Denim is versatile. Use denim for more than only one look; pair it with different items of clothing and jewellery to get the most out of your denim clothes. Create your own personal style.

- Always wear a style of denim that is comfortable and flattering. Wear it because it makes you look good, not because it is the latest fashion.

Chapter 13: The 50 Best Fashion Tips of All Time

Now that we have worked through all the information, it is time to sift through the information and compile a list to carry with you. With this list you will be able to identify at first glance what the 50 most important fashion tips are.

1. Show skin strategically.
You should know where and when to show some skin for a more sexy look and how not to do it. Bare your skin only at one place to create emphasis. If you are wearing a mini skirt, do not wear a low cleavage shirt. It is better to keep a certain sense of mystery if you want to look stylish.

2. Have a collection of classic white shirts.
A white shirt is one of the items that should feature in every wardrobe. You can wear a white shirt with anything and you can wear it anywhere. Unfortunately, this can lead to faster wear and tear of your shirt and make it look yellow sooner. Be prepared for this by stocking up on white shirts. Always keep a spare or two at hand for emergencies.

3. Use bright colors as accessories.
Give your neutral colors a boost by adding shoes, handbags or jewellery in bright colors. It is good to have clothes in navy, black, gray or camel as it is versatile and safe to wear. Avoid being stuck in a dull rut by spicing up your outfit with trendy bold colors.

4. Buy multiples of one style.
This may sound strange, but if you find a style that flatters you and makes you look good, buy the style in various lengths and colors. There is a saying of "if the shoe fits, buy a pair in each color!"

5. Know the combination of materials for stretch.
This may also sound strange, but certain materials combined in specific ways, creates a better fit than what other creates. If you are looking for the best-fit t-shirt to fit your form, buy a t-shirt that is 95% cotton and 5% Lycra spandex. Jeans should be 2% Lycra spandex to fit properly and keep their shape.

6. Adjust hems of pants and skirts.
Hems of your pants should be ½ inch to ¾ of an inch from the floor to fit with your shoe. It is therefore important to have two pairs of the same pants, one to wear with high-heeled shoes and a pair to wear with ballet flats.

7. Add a scarf.
A scarf is one of the most popular accessories currently. It is classic and has been around for a very long time and it is projected to stay on the list for a long time still to come. Keep a scarf handy to transform a plain outfit to interesting.

8. Carry a clutch bag with a chain.
Holding on to a clutch bag at a cocktail event may look very elegant, but it is very unpractical at times. Every person who has ever tried to hold on to her clutch bag, holding a drink and trying to taste some of the snacks, will know how tricky this can be. Go for a clutch bag with an elegant chain to wear over your shoulder. It will add comfort without compromising style.

9. Wear and care of your clothing.
Clothing needs to last you a while. You do not want to buy a new item every other day because of damage to the previous item. You also do not want to spend ages to iron your clothes because your item of clothing crinkles fast. Check the labels of clothing for caring instructions to see if the item is high maintenance. Care properly for your clothes to extend its lifespan.

10. Love your body shape.
You were born with a specific body shape and you have to live with that shape. Come to terms with it and accept your body shape. Learn which styles flatter you and which styles to avoid and make the best of the body you have.

11. Do shopping with a list.
Create a list of the key items you already own. The list will remind you of what works with your current wardrobe and what you should avoid.

It will save you time to know what to buy and save you money to not buy items you do not need.

12. Be prepared for the dressing room.
When shopping for a certain garment, take all the items you will need with you to get a true reflection of how the outfit will look before you buy it. Take your high heels with you, the bag you plan to use, your lipstick and your planned accessories. It will save you a lot of frustration later.

13. All over view.
After you are dressed, view yourself from every angle to make sure everything is perfect and in place. It can be a very long outing if you discover afterwards that some body parts are accentuated negatively.

14. The true size of your denim.
When you buy a new denim and you are unsure of your size, rather go for the smaller size. Denims stretch when you wear it, so buying a size smaller will end up looking better than a larger size that will stretch and look baggy.

15. Sort out your closet.
When looking at your wardrobe, you need to be able to see all your clothes at one glance. Throw out what you do not need and leave only your key items. Donate the clothes you do not wear to charity or to someone who will need the clothes more than you do.

16. Necklace layered.
Layer necklaces of different lengths for a dramatic effect. You can use necklaces made of the same material, or combine different types to create contrast.

17. Inspect linings.
The lining of clothes is a good indication of the quality of the garment. An item of good quality will be carefully and precisely sewn on the inside.

18. Be open-minded.

You will never know how good an item looks on you unless you try it on. When fitting clothes in a dressing room, take an item with you that you would not normally consider. You may surprise yourself at how well it suits you.

19. Be loyal to a good designer.
If you find an item of clothing that flatters you and make you look gorgeous, chances are that there will be an item in the next range that will be just as flattering. Once you have found such a designer, be loyal to him as you are almost certain to have success with his clothing line.

20. Wear nude pumps.
If you are uncertain of which shoes to wear, select a pair of nude pumps. It will flatter any skin tone and outfit and will elongate your legs.

21. White clothes rules.
If you plan to wear a white garment, stand in bright light to see the effect of your garment. White items tend to be more see-through when you are in light, so take that into consideration when you get dressed.

22. Stripes.
Wear clothing with stripes for a fun alternative way to dress over the weekend or holidays. It is trendy and youthful and looks great when worn with solid colours.

23. Button up.
Remove buttons that looks cheap and makes your jacket look cheap. Sew some stylish buttons onto your jacket to give it an instant upgrade.

24. Coat is the word.
Jackets and coats play a very important role in the overall look of your outfit. In the cold months, your coat may be the only item other people see, so make it worth your while and buy an exciting and great fitting coat.

25. Leopard prints.

Each person should own at least one item with a leopard print. It can be a handbag, a pair of shoes, a belt or a scarf. Whichever you choose, make sure it is a key item in your wardrobe.

26. Mixing of prints.
Be careful and selective when mixing prints. Rather stay with one print if you are not one hundred percent certain you can wear the look successfully.

27. Go wild with color.
Add bright colours to neutral colors to liven up your outfit. If you are more daring, mix bold colors together. Work with a color wheel to combine colors that are next to each other for harmony, or colors opposite each other for a dramatic look. Stay with colors that you like and that looks good on you.

28. Accentuate.
You only need one piece of accessory that is jaw dropping to accentuate an outfit that is a showstopper in its own right. Anything more will be overdoing it.

29. Vintage items.
Vintage is not always vintage. Sometimes it is just old and will make you look older. Be selective when wearing an item that you think is vintage and ask for a second opinion.

30. Rethink a bargain.
A bargain is only a bargain if you really like it and plan to wear it often. Paying $100 for an item that is usually $200 may be a bargain, but it is a waste of money if you are not going to wear it.

31. The wonders of a thick waistband.
If you need to slim down your waist a bit, wear a thick belt or waistband. It will make your waist look slimmer, but it will also accentuate your upper body to create an hourglass image.

32. The casual jacket.
Besides your tailored jacket for formal events, you should also own a casual jacket to wear down over weekends or holidays or just enjoying

time with friends. Leather jackets or army jackets are good candidates for casual days.

33. Menswear.
If you are planning to make a statement in menswear, wear it correctly with a pinstripe pants, elegant shirt and even a waistcoat. Finish off the look with a feminine touch by adding your favourite lipstick and a pair of high heels.

34. Alter with a tailor.
Have your clothes altered to achieve a proper fit. It flatters your figure and improves the look of your clothes. Find a good local tailor you can trust that can do alterations and customise your clothes. It will be worth it when you see the looks of admiration on other peoples' faces.

35. Look for revamped classics.
Many of your favorite classics are now available with an all new twist. Look out for trench coats that now come in silk, tote bags in camouflage motifs and other remade classics.

36. Undercover stories.
Do not under estimate the power of a well fitted t-shirt bra. T-shirt material can be very unforgiving and accentuate what least need to be accentuated. Find a t-shirt bra that gives you confidence and proper shape.

37. Surprise!
Never be predictable. Add an interesting touch to your outfit that will surprise people. Add the unexpected to make a bold statement.

38. Jewellery with a twist.
Combine certain jewellery pieces to make an interesting new piece. Wrap a necklace around your wrist and wear it a bracelet. Wear rings on a chain as pendants. Combine a brooch and a chain to form a new necklace. The possibilities are endless when you use your imagination.

39. Accessorise!
Not enough can be said about the importance of accessories to transform an outfit. With a limited budget you can always buy a new focus piece of jewellery that you can wear with many different outfits.

40. Pack a style emergency kit.

Fashion emergencies can occur at any time and any place. Be prepared for all the unforeseen emergencies. A few necessities are:

- Eraser pen to quickly get rid of wine stains on white clothes

- A lint brush to brush off fluff on a coat or jersey

- Safety pins

- Double-sided tape for hems or a strapless bodice

- clips to keep bra straps in place

- A makeup sponge to remove stains caused by deodorant

41. Perfect loose and tight fit.

Combine a baggy shirt with stretch jeans. Wear an A-line shirt or mini with leggings. It is very feminine and very trendy and suitable for almost all body types.

42. Spiced your little black dress.

Wear a trendy jacket or sexy boots with sheer stockings with your favorite little black dress. This tip works well when your dress is styled in a simple way. The additional accessories will add much needed pizzazz to your overall look.

43. Be a stud muffin.

Wear studs as jewellery piece. It is subtle and versatile and comes with various gems in. It goes with any outfit and will never take away the focus from another piece of jewellery.

44. Always dress to impress.

It is not necessary to dress up everywhere you go, but at least dress in a manner that make you feel comfortable and confident. For a chic and universal trendy look, wear a jacket or cashmere shirt with leggings, a scarf and a pair of ballet flat. Add a scarf and you are ready to face the world.

45. Rise and fall.
Jeans and other trousers are cut in various ways to accommodate every shape and size of body. Choose jeans and pants that fit properly and have the correct rise and width to flatter your body. Modern pants are made to balance out flaws and add accent to positive areas.

46. Notes on cashmere.
Good quality cashmere is thick and has a dense gauge. Cashmere should be slightly elastic and return to its original shape after being stretched. The best cashmere is woven in Scotland and Italy.

47. Snap your look.
If you wore a gorgeous combination of clothes and received many compliments on your look, take a photo of that outfit. It will work as a quick reference guide when you urgently need to find a stunning outfit on short notice.

48. Make your body look good, the rest will follow.
You should always dress to flatter your body shape. If your body is in balance and harmony, you will have the added benefit of also looking more youthful.

49. Dress age appropriately, though.
What looked good on you when you were a teenager will not be suitable anymore. You had your time of being young and free; give your children the opportunity now to dress like teenagers.

50. Slimming in a shoe.
Pumps with thick soles and ultra high heels will make any ankle look slimmer. D'Orsay pumps are ultra flattering and a must for every shoe collection.

Chapter 14: Additional Tips on How to Dress to Look Young

Now that we have covered all the areas regarding style and fashion and how to wear it for a youthful look, let us summarise what we have discussed.

What every short man should know

Being short does not mean you should have a bad posture or you may slouch. Sit up straight with your back straight. Keep your posture proud and your head high.

Wear a shorter hairstyle so your neck and shoulders can show. This creates a longer look, while hiding your neck behind your hair will make your neck look shorter, ultimately making you look shorter.

With the risk of sounding superficial: Try to keep in shape. A trim body will look less short than a rounded body will.

When shopping for clothes, choose pants or shirts with vertical stripes to create an illusion of length. Avoid shirts with checks or plaids. Wear a pants and shirt of the same color. When you wear two different colours, it breaks the silhouette into blocks, creating a shorter illusion. Short men should create the illusion of an uninterrupted straight vertical line.

Wear darker shades of clothes to make you look slimmer, especially if you have an endomorph body shape. Always make sure your clothes are well fitted. Your pants should cover your socks completely and end a little lower than where your shoe starts. Your pants should however not be too long or it will inevitably make you look too short for your pants.

Choose shoes that add length. These are usually the bulkier shoes with thicker soles and ankle boot-type shoes. It will also make your feet look bigger.

What every tall man should know

Tall men face different challenges than short men. It may even be more difficult for them to find suitable clothes than it is for short men. Many times when buying clothes from a department store, you are faced with the problem that the pants are too short, the shirt cannot tuck into your pants properly or it fits too tight.

Buy your clothes from either speciality stores, or from department stores that includes a section for tall men. If you do not have that option, it is necessary that you have you have your pants or shirts lengthened by either tailors or the dry-cleaners.

When shopping, look for clothes that do not add extra length to your already tall frame. Choose shirts with blocks or horizontal lines. Wear separate colors for your pants and shirt to break the tall effect. By breaking your frame into visible blocks, you will appear shorter. Wear wider cuffs and lapels to create width.

What every large man should know

One of the biggest mistakes larger men make, no pun intended, is to wear baggy clothes, thinking it will cover up their extra size. This could not be further from the truth. The secret is to wear well -fitted clothes to balance out your flaws, rather that covering it up.

You will need to wear clothes that create a slimmer illusion and avoid adding additional bulk. Choose clothes in darker colours to slim you down. Avoid patterned shirts and choose vertical lines instead.

Choose pants with a loose fit, but not baggy and avoid wearing tight fitting pants. Stay clear of pants with pleats as it will draw attention to your waist and pelvic area, creating a bigger illusion, instead of smaller. Always make sure your pants are well-fitted.

When you need to wear a blazer, choose a single breasted blazer. The double breasted option will only make your waist and shoulders look broader and draw unnecessary attention to your waist.

What every athletic man should know

If you are an athletic built man, you probably have a well-shaped upper body which is larger than your lower body. When buying clothes, this may present a problem you do not want to hide the result of your hard work and training under baggy clothes. Buying a large shirt to fit properly over your broad shoulders will result in the bottom of the shirt hanging formless at your well-sculptured waist.

It is almost a given that for an extreme athletic built male, the most obvious option is to have your clothes tailor made. Again, not every person has the budget and luxury for such an option. You will then need to select clothes that will take attention away from your broad shoulders and add attention to your slimmer waist.

For long sleeved shirts, choose a style with wide cuffs that will draw attention to your waist. A jacket should be buttoned to add the necessary width. Choose vest type shirt in the summer. The strappy vest will expose your shoulders without adding extra width, while the body of the shirt will create width at your waist.

Pants should be also well-fitted. Try a pair of pants with pleats to create width to balance out your shoulders, but will look slim enough to balance out with your hips that are wider than your legs.

Choose bulky shoes to create height if needed and to make your feet look bigger. The bigger shoes will balance out your hips.

For women: rules regarding makeup

Determine your skin season and under tones and apply makeup accordingly. The most important rule is to apply makeup and still look natural. Make-up should enhance your natural beauty; it should not be worn as a mask.

Apply makeup in a subtle manner. Accentuate your eye color by applying an appropriate color of eye shadow. People should notice your eyes, not your eye shadow. The moment someone tells you that you are wearing nice eye shadow and only after that notices your eyes, then you know you are wearing too much eye shadow.

The same applies to the rest of your makeup. Your cheeks should have a healthy glow, not look like a picture from a grade one coloring book. Your lips should be soft and kissable. The latest trend is to wear a colored lip gloss or one coat color lasting lipstick. There is no need any more to wear three coats of lipstick for it to last longer. Lip liner is still important to prevent your lip color from "bleeding", but wear a liner in a neutral color, or a color that matches your lipstick exactly.

The rule for makeup is therefore: less is more. You want to go out your front door looking like a princess and not like a pizza.

Shed twenty pounds

This rule can mean physically losing the weight, or it can be to virtually losing the weight by dressing to look slimmer. Let us discuss both scenarios.

- Physical weight loss

Firstly, you should only attempt to shed twenty pound if you have an excess of twenty ponds to shed. Loosing unwanted weight not only makes you look and feel better, it is also healthy. Being overweight has serious health risks such as diabetes and heart complications. By losing the weight, you will most certainly improve your health.

The first steps to take to lose weight, is to exercise more and to eat less. What it comes down to, in simple terms, is that you should burn more energy than what you consume.

Since this guide is not about weight loss and it is not so easy for everybody as it may sound, so speak to your health practitioner may give you advice on how to effectively lose weight and how to maintain it once you have reached your goal.

- Virtual weight loss

If you need to look twenty pounds lighter for an important function you have in a day or two, you most certainly won't have time to shed that weight. Not safely, at least. Your second option is then to select specific items of clothing and wear it strategically to create an illusion of being slimmer.

Determine your body shape and wear clothes that balance out imperfections and accentuate your good features. Wear accessories to complement your outfit and add additional emphasis where needed. It will make you look good and flawless, but it will also make you feel invincible.

Let go of outdated clothes

Yesterday is gone and the past belongs in the past. So does outdated clothes. Hanging on to outdated styles will not create a youthful appearance, in fact, it will declare to the outside world in which era you grew up. We do not want that, do we? I do not think so.

If you have to cling to your outdated clothes and still need to wear them, match them up with more modern pieces of clothing and accessories to authenticate your style. Spice up your clothes by wearing it with a funky jacket or stylish shoes and add some trendy jewellery. If you cannot successfully incorporate old with new, your sentimental clothes should rather be packed up and kept in the attic along with your photos of days gone by.

Smile constantly throughout the day

This is the best fashion advice that you will ever receive. Be positive and be yourself. No amount of fashion and make-up can recreate your personality and self-confidence. Be friendly and be a pleasure for the people around you.

Always keep on smiling!